WEIGHT LOSS JUICING RECIPE FOR BEGINNERS.

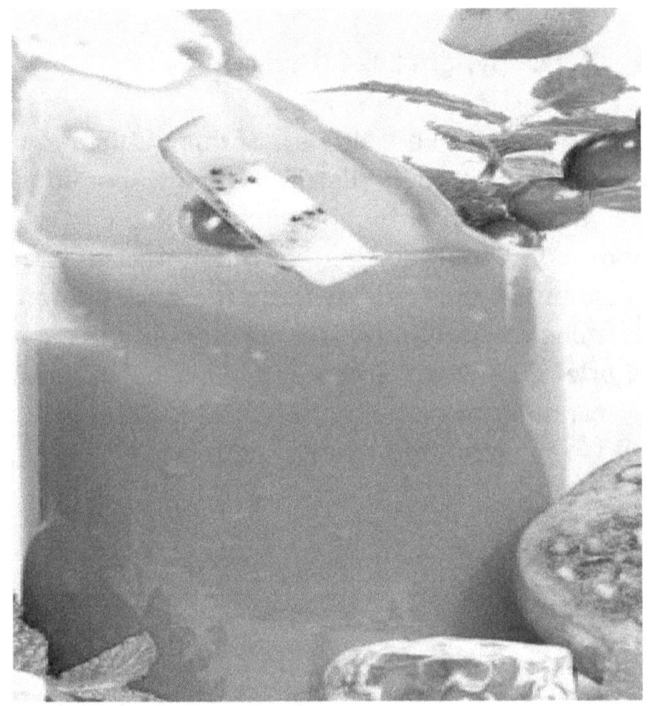

A tasty juicing blend for vitality and weight loss.

Hudson Alexis

TABLE OF CONTENT

INTRODUCTION

For overweight individuals and fitness lovers, juicing has shown to be a very successful weight loss strategy. A great and healthful way to start your weight loss journey is with nutritious, freshly squeezed juices. Juicing encourages you to stay hydrated and provides your body with the vitamins, minerals, and antioxidants it need. Enjoy a variety of fruits, veggies, and herbs in a delightful and convenient way.

Novice juicers should grasp the basics and approach weight loss with a well-rounded plan when they first begin. Decreasing your body weight and satisfying your palate can be achieved by selecting the right ingredients and combinations. In a healthy lifestyle, juicing can be a terrific complement to regular exercise and a balanced diet. However, it is not a weight loss help on its own.

Aim to incorporate low-calorie fruits and vegetables into your meals, such as celery, apples, berries, and cucumbers, as well as low-calorie fruits like grapefruits, spinach, and kale. These nutrients are low in calories and high in vitamins, minerals, and fibre. Consider including digestive and metabolic-boosting herbs like ginger or mint for further benefits.

Remember to visit a qualified dietitian or get medical advice before starting any weight loss regimen, including juicing. Apart from providing you with a well-balanced juice diet that effectively aids in your weight loss goals, they can also provide you with customised advice based on your individual requirements.

Integrating weight loss juicing into your overall healthy lifestyle may benefit you in the form of increased hydration, increased nutritional intake, and potentially even faster weight loss. With a delicious and nutritious meal plan, you may start your weight loss journey by selecting your favourite flavours and experimenting with new combinations.

CHAPTER 1

THE BASIC

What is Juicing?

Juicing is the process of taking the liquid out of fruits and vegetables while discarding the fibre and pulp. Juice is a drink that's usually drunk for its high nutritional content and possible health advantages. A range of appliances, like blenders and juicers, can be used for juicing; these devices grind or crush the produce to extract the juice. The resulting juice can be a handy way to include a variety of fruits and vegetables in one's diet, and it is frequently high in vitamins, minerals, and antioxidants. Juicing has become popular among those who want to follow a cleansing program or enhance their vitamin intake.

Juicing has advantages over consuming raw fruit and vegetables.

Juicing is the process of removing the pulp Fand just keeping the juice from fruits and vegetables. Produce-derived vitamins, minerals, and phytonutrients are concentrated in this liquid, called juice. A blender or a juicer machine can be used for juicing.

The advantages of juicing consist of:

1. Better absorption of nutrients: Juicing reduces the need for the body to break down fibre, which makes it easier for nutrients to be absorbed.

2.Increased consumption of fruits and vegetables: Juicing offers a practical approach to eat more fruits and vegetables at once.

3. Improved hydration: Juices assist the body stay hydrated because of their high water content.

4. Easy and quick digestion: By eliminating the fibre, the body can absorb the nutrients more quickly, giving off a rapid energy boost.

5. Variety of Flavors: Consuming a wide range of fruits and vegetables is made delightful by the limitless flavour combinations that may be created by juicing.

However, there are advantages to consuming fruits and vegetables uncooked as well:

1. *Dietary fibre:* Fibre from whole fruits and vegetables aids in blood sugar regulation, aids in digestion, and supports a healthy weight.

2. *Satiety*: Chewing whole fruits and vegetables prolongs the time it takes to feel full, which can aid in controlling portion sizes and weight.

3. *Dental health*: Chewing fibrous food encourages the production of saliva, which supports good dental hygiene.

4. *Slow release of nutrients*: Whole fruits and vegetables include fibre, which reduces the rate at which sugars enter the bloodstream and avoids blood sugar spikes.

In summary, eating raw fruits and vegetables offers the advantages of dietary fibre, satiety, oral health, and a slower release of nutrients, whereas juicing offers a concentrated intake of nutrients and facilitates quick absorption. A balanced diet that includes whole produce as well as juiced produce can have many positive health effects.

Juicing to Remove Toxins

Juicing detoxification, sometimes referred to as juice cleaning or juice fasting, is a method where you spend a set amount of time ingesting only freshly squeezed fruit and vegetable juices. The idea is to overload your body with nutrient-rich drinks while providing a vacation for your digestive system.

Juicing a range of fruits and vegetables to make a concentrated drink is the substitute for solid foods, processed drinks, and stimulants during a juice detox. This procedure reduces the amount of dietary fibre consumed while facilitating simple absorption of vitamins, minerals, and antioxidants.

Proponents of detoxification by juicing assert that it can aid in the removal of toxins, enhance overall well-being, improve digestion, increase energy, encourage weight loss, and rejuvenate the skin. It's crucial to remember that there is little scientific proof to back up these assertions, and the liver and kidneys are the main organs used by the body's natural detoxification process.

Consult a healthcare provider before beginning a juice cleanse because extended juice fasting can result in vitamin deficits and other health hazards.

Tips for Juicing:

- ***Include a Variety***: Aim for a diverse selection of fruits and vegetables to ensure a broad spectrum of nutrients.
- ***Moderation is Key***: While juicing can be a healthy addition to a balanced diet, it should

not replace whole fruits and vegetables entirely.

- **Mindful Ingredient Selection**: Be mindful of the sugar content in fruits and consider adding leafy greens and vegetables to balance sweetness and enhance nutritional value.
- **Drink Immediately**: Freshly juiced beverages are most nutritious when consumed immediately, as exposure to air and light can lead to nutrient degradation.

In conclusion, juicing can be a convenient way to boost nutrient intake and support hydration, but it should be approached with moderation and a balanced perspective. It's essential to consider individual health goals, dietary needs, and potential drawbacks before incorporating juicing into one's routine.

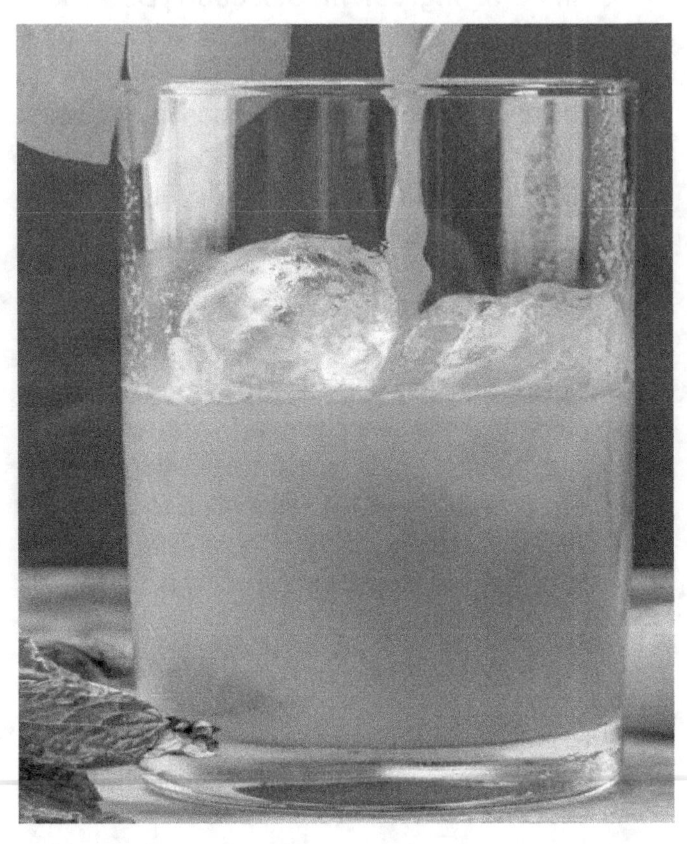

CHAPTER 2

FRUIT

Fruit refers to the mature ovary of a flowering plant that typically contains seeds. Fruits are usually consumed for their sweet or savoury taste and are a rich source of various nutrients, including vitamins, minerals, and dietary fibre. They come in a wide variety of shapes, sizes, colours, and flavours.

Some popular examples of fruits include:

1. *Apples*: They come in various types, such as Granny Smith, Red Delicious, and Gala, and are known for their crisp texture and sweet or tart taste.

2. *Oranges*: Known for their bright orange colour and juicy flesh, oranges are a rich source of vitamin C.

3. *Bananas*: They are one of the most commonly consumed fruits worldwide and are known for their creamy texture and sweet taste.

4. *Strawberries*: These small, red fruits are known for their sweet and tangy flavour and are often enjoyed fresh or used in desserts.

5. *Grapes*: Available in different colours like green, red, or purple, grapes are often consumed fresh or used to make wine or raisins.

6. *Watermelons*: They have a refreshing and juicy flesh, usually eaten as a summer treat.

7. *Pineapples*: These tropical fruits have a sweet and tangy taste and are known for their spiky outer skin and juicy yellow flesh.

8. *Mangoes*: Considered the "king of fruits," mangoes are known for their sweet, tropical flavour and are popular in many cuisines.

9. *Kiwis*: These small, green fruits have a fuzzy brown exterior and a tangy, sweet flavour.

10. *Blueberries*: These small, dark-blue berries are packed with antioxidants and are often enjoyed fresh or used in baking.

These are just a few examples, and there are many more types of fruits available with their own unique characteristics and flavours.

CHAPTER 3

VEGETABLES

Vegetables are a vital component of a balanced diet and are important for preserving general health and wellbeing. They are abundant in vital vitamins, minerals, fibre, and health-promoting antioxidants.

Vegetables are significant for the following main reasons:

1. *High in nutrients:* Vegetables are high in vital nutrients, including dietary fibre, potassium, magnesium, and iron, as well as vitamins A, C, K, and folate. These nutrients are essential for sustaining good health, assisting with different body processes, and avoiding nutrient shortages.

2. *Disease prevention*: It is well known that vegetables can prevent disease. Their high antioxidant content and low calorie content help shield the body from chronic illnesses like heart disease, certain cancers, and age-related macular degeneration.

3. *Fibre content:* Rich in dietary fibre, vegetables facilitate proper digestion, support gut health, and ward against constipation. By promoting satiety and lowering the likelihood of overeating, fibre also aids in weight management.

4. *Hydration*: The high water content of many vegetables contributes to the body's ability to stay properly hydrated. Maintaining hydration is crucial for a number of biological processes, such as regulating body temperature, transporting nutrients, and lubricating joints.

5. *Weight management*: Eating more vegetables will help you maintain a healthy weight. They are high in fibre and low in calories, which helps to maintain a healthy weight by increasing satiety and controlling appetite.

6. *Digestive health:* Vegetables' high fibre content encourages regular bowel movements and guards against digestive illnesses like haemorrhoids, diverticulosis, and constipation.

7. *General health and vitality*: Eating veggies on a regular basis has been associated with better general health and vitality. They are a great option for fulfilling daily nutritional needs while keeping a healthy weight because of their nutrient density and low calorie content.

Varieties of Vegetables

1. *Green leafy vegetables.*

- Lettuce, Swiss chard, Arugula, Collard greens, Bok choy, Spinach, Kale

2. *Cruciferous Vegetables*:

- Brussels sprouts, cauliflower, broccoli, cabbage, radishes, turnips, and kale.

3. *Vegetables with roots:*

- Carrots, potatoes, sweet potatoes, beets, radishes, parsnips, and turnips.

4. *Vegetables with Allium:*
- Garlic, Onions, Shallots, Leeks , Scallions, Chives.

5. *Vegetables that are Nightshade:*
- Tomatoes, Peppers (chilli and bell peppers), Eggplants, Potatoes.

6. *Squash and Gourds:*
- Cucumbers, Watermelon, Pumpkin, Zucchini, Butternut squash, Acorn squash, Spaghetti squash.

7. *Legumes*:
- legumes, chickpeas, kidney beans, black beans, lentils, green beans, and soybeans.

8. *Brassica Vegetables:*
- Kohlrabi, Chinese cabbage, broccoli, cauliflower, Brussels sprouts, and cabbage.

9. *Edible tubers:*
sweet potatoes, yams, taro, Jerusalem artichokes, jicama, and cassava.

10. *Additional Vegetables*:
- Celery, Cucumbers, Corn , Asparagus, Mushrooms, Artichokes, Okra.

Every vegetable has a different nutritional profile and can be cooked and consumed in different ways.

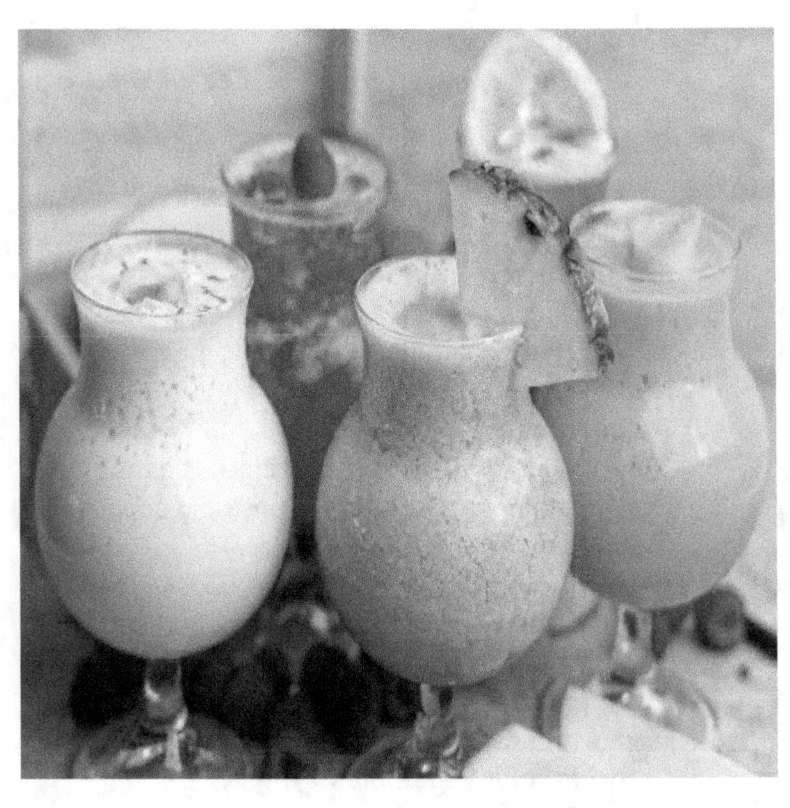

CHAPTER 4

JUICING TO REDUCE WEIGHT

Juicing's many advantages have made it more and more popular as a weight loss strategy. Here are several main justifications for why juicing may be beneficial for losing weight:

1. ***Nutrient Density:*** By juicing fruits and vegetables, you can ingest a concentrated amount of vital nutrients. Juices that have been freshly squeezed are high in vitamins, minerals, and antioxidants that can help with weight loss while also promoting general health and wellbeing.
2. ***Portion Control:*** Juicing offers a filling and healthy beverage in a portion-controlled serving size, which can assist with portion control. You can cut calories overall and establish the calorie deficit required for weight loss by swapping out a high-calorie meal with a low-calorie juice.
3. ***Hydration***: Maintaining hydration is essential for losing weight. Because most fruits and vegetables used in juicing have a high water content, juicing encourages hydration. Drinking enough water helps improve metabolism, facilitate better digestion, and assist the body's natural detoxifying processes.
4. ***Increased Fibre Intake***: Although the liquid from fruits and vegetables is extracted mostly during juicing, some fibre is still present in the juice.

Because it stimulates feelings of fullness, controls blood sugar, and aids in proper digestion, fibre is crucial for weight loss. But it's important to remember that much of the insoluble fibre in whole fruits and vegetables is lost during the juicing process.

5. ***Detoxification***: By giving the body an abundance of antioxidants and phytochemicals, juicing can help with the detoxification process. By boosting the liver's detoxification processes and neutralising toxins, these substances can promote weight reduction by increasing metabolic efficiency.

6. *Variety and Taste:* You can juice a wide variety of fruits and vegetables to experience a wide range of flavours and nutrients. This diversity helps minimise boredom and encourage long-term adherence to a weight loss strategy by making healthy eating more pleasurable and sustainable.

Even though juicing can help with weight loss, it's crucial to keep in mind that it shouldn't completely replace full foods or a balanced diet. Juices are to be consumed in conjunction with a balanced diet rich in complex carbs, lean proteins, and healthy fats. Before making any major dietary changes, it's also advisable to speak with a medical expert or certified dietician, particularly if you have underlying medical concerns or are taking medication.

CHAPTER 5

PUDDING FOR SUCCESS

Juicing is a common practice that involves using fresh produce to extract the juice, which is packed with nutrients, to support vitality. Juicing is said by many to offer a concentrated form of vitamins, minerals, and antioxidants that can support general health and vigour. Although adding extra fruits and vegetables to your diet by juicing can be handy, there are a few things to keep in mind when doing so.

1. *Select a range of fruits and vegetables:* In order to get the most nutritional value out of your juices, incorporate a variety of fruits and vegetables. It's beneficial to have a variety of fruits and vegetables since they provide different amounts of vitamins, minerals, and phytochemicals. Nutrient-dense leafy greens such as Swiss chard, kale, and spinach are great options.

2. *Fresh and organic vegetables:* To guarantee that you're limiting your exposure to pesticides and optimising the nutritional worth of the contents, use fresh, organic produce wherever possible. When it comes to fruits and vegetables, fresh produce usually has more nutrients than produce that has been kept in storage for longer.

3. *Make use of a high-quality juicer:* Make an investment in a juicer that efficiently extracts juice from the fruits and vegetables of your choice. When compared to high-speed centrifugal juicers, cold-press juicers are frequently chosen since they run at slower speeds, conserving more nutrients and enzymes in the juice.

4. *Use moderation:* Juicing has its advantages, but it's crucial to keep in mind that it shouldn't take the place of full fruits and vegetables in your diet. Dietary fibre, which is crucial for healthy digestion and general well-being, is eliminated during the juicer process. Fibre increases satiety and slows down the body's absorption of sugar. Juice should therefore be consumed sparingly and in conjunction with a well-balanced diet.

5. *Drink juice right away:* Juices that are freshly produced are at their most nutrient-dense when they are drunk right away. Heat, air, and light exposure can cause the juice's nutritional value to decline. If you must preserve juice for later use, store it in airtight containers in the refrigerator and attempt to finish it within a day or two.

6. *Think about adding herbs and spices*: You can experiment with adding herbs and spices to your juices to improve their flavour and possible health benefits. Herbs like mint and basil can offer a refreshing touch, while anti-inflammatory qualities like ginger and turmeric are also present.

7. *Pay attention to your body*: Since each person is different, what suits one person may not suit another. Keep an eye on your body's reaction to juicing. Before making big dietary changes, it's always a good idea to speak with a healthcare provider if you have any specific health conditions or notice any negative affects.

To ensure you're getting a well-rounded and balanced diet, remember that while juicing can be a component of a healthy lifestyle, it's crucial to eat a range of entire foods, including fruits, vegetables, whole grains, lean proteins, and healthy fats.

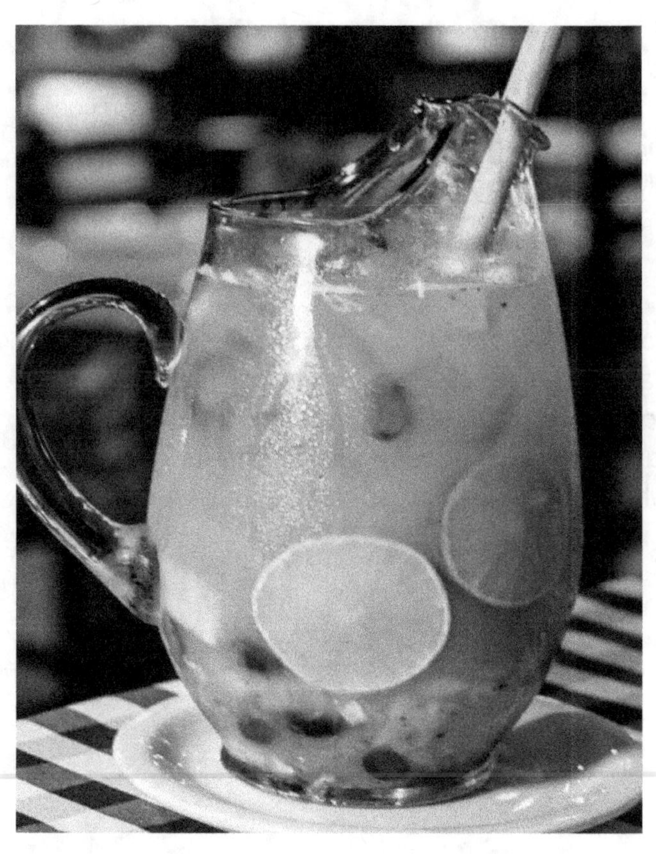

CHAPTER 6

VARIOUS FRUIT BASED JUICE

EARLY MELON BOOST

A melon boost in the morning sounds good. One way to get ready is to whip up a tasty smoothie with melon. I'll give you a basic recipe here:

Ingredients:
- 1/2 cup Greek yoghourt
- 1 cup diced melon (such as watermelon, cantaloupe, or honeydew)
- Half a cup of ordinary or coconut water
- One tablespoon (optional) of honey or another sweetener
- Ice cubes, if desired

Instructions:
1. First, get your melon ready. Cut the melon into small pieces after removing the seeds and rind.
2. Fill a blender with the chopped melon, Greek yoghourt, and coconut water (or ordinary water).
3. You can add honey or another preferred sweetener if you'd like it sweeter. Certain melons are inherently sweet enough that you don't need to do this step.

4. Process all the ingredients in a blender until a creamy, smooth consistency is reached. You may also add a few ice cubes and blend them in if you want your smoothie to be colder.

5. After the smoothie is blended, taste it and adjust the sweetness or thickness to suit your tastes. If necessary, you can add extra liquid, yoghourt, or honey.

6. Transfer the smoothie into a glass, and if preferred, top with a melon slice or a sprig of mint.

7. Savour your melon boost in the morning! Any leftovers can be chilled for later use.

To make your smoothie unique, feel free to try out different melon varieties and add other fruits. Melons are a fantastic option for a morning boost because they are hydrating, refreshing, and high in vitamins.

APPLE CIDER JUICE

Because of its high vitamin content and low calorie content, apple celery juice can be an excellent supplement to any weight loss regimen. Celery and apples are both high in fibre and low in calories, which can help you feel filled for longer periods of time and consume less calories overall. They also include high levels of antioxidants, vitamins, and minerals, all of which are good for general health.

Easy recipe for celery and apple juice:

Components:
- Two apples
- Four celery stalks
- Water (optional, for diluting)

Directions:
1. Thoroughly wash the apples and celery stalks to get rid of any residue or dirt.
2. Cut out the apple cores and seeds. Peel them if you'd like, or leave the skin on for more nutrients.
3. To make it easier to juice, chop the apples and celery into small pieces.
4. Put the apple and celery pieces through a juicer to get the juice out of them. Make sure you adhere to the directions that came with your juicer.
5. You can dilute the juice to your preferred taste by adding a small bit of water if it's too powerful or concentrated.
6. Make sure the liquid is well combined by giving it a good stir.
7. Transfer the apple-celery juice into a glass or other container, and serve immediately!

Don't forget to drink the juice right away for the most flavour and nutritious value. In the event that you lack a juicer, you can still extract the juice using a blender and filter it through cheesecloth or a fine-mesh sieve to eliminate any debris.

KIWI ORANGE JUICE

Because kiwi orange juice is low in calories and high in vital nutrients, it can be a delightful and healthful supplement to your diet plan for weight loss. Excellent providers of vitamin C, dietary fibre, and antioxidants that can improve general health and help with weight management are kiwis and oranges. This is a basic recipe for making orange juice from kiwis:

Ingredients:
- Two oranges
- Two ripe kiwis
- Water (to be diluted, optional)

Direction:
1. Peel the oranges and kiwis first. Take off the white pith from the oranges because it can make the juice more bitter.
2. Make sure the oranges and kiwis are seedless by chopping them into little pieces.
3. Transfer the orange and kiwi pieces to a juicer or blender.
4. Process the fruit in a blender or juicer until the consistency is smooth.
5. You can add water to thin the juice to the right consistency if you think it's too thick.
6. Immediately serve the juice by pouring it into a glass.
7. For extra visual appeal, you can, if you'd like, garnish the juice with a slice of orange or kiwi.

Remember that maintaining a balanced diet and getting regular exercise are crucial for good weight control, even though kiwi orange juice can be a healthy supplement to your weight loss efforts. Additionally, for individualised guidance based on your unique dietary requirements and medical concerns, speak with a healthcare provider or a qualified dietitian.

CILANTRO, BANANA JUICE, AND STRAWBERRY

You can include some healthy and delicious cilantro strawberry banana juice to your weight loss regimen. While cilantro offers a distinct flavour and certain health advantages, strawberries, bananas, and other fruits are high in vital nutrients and low in calories. This is an easy recipe to create strawberry-banana juice with cilantro:

Ingredients:
 - 1 ripe banana
- 1 cup fresh strawberries
- One-fourth cup of fresh cilantro
- One cup of water, or coconut water; adjust amount to desired consistency.
- Ice cubes, if desired

Direction:
1. Clean the strawberries, cut off the stems, and cut them into quarters or halves.

2. After peeling, chop the banana into small pieces.
3. Give the cilantro leaves a good rinse to get rid of any remaining dirt or debris.
4. Put the banana, cilantro leaves, strawberries, and water or coconut water in a blender.
5. Process the ingredients at a high speed until a smooth consistency is reached.
6. To make the juice colder and more energising, feel free to add a few ice cubes. Repeatedly blend until the ice cubes are well combined and smashed.
7. If preferred, add a natural sweetener, like as stevia or honey, to the juice to modify its sweetness.
8. Transfer the juice into a glass and start serving right away.

Remember that portion management and total nutritional balance are more important than any one ingredient in a weight loss strategy, even if cilantro strawberry banana juice can be a nutritious addition. For optimal effects, include this juice in a nutrient-dense, well-rounded diet along with frequent exercise. Seeking advice from a medical practitioner or qualified dietitian is always a good idea if you have any specific dietary concerns or health conditions.

JUICE OF ORANGE, CARROT AND GINGER

Fresh oranges, carrots, and ginger are combined to make orange carrot ginger juice, a hydrating and nourishing drink. It's a well-liked option for anyone looking for a tasty and nutritious beverage. Here's a basic recipe for orange carrot ginger juice that you can follow:

Ingredients:
 - 1 inch of fresh ginger
- 4 medium-sized oranges
- 4 medium-sized carrots

Directions:
1. Peel and cut the oranges into segments.
2. To make juicing easier, peel and cut the carrots into smaller pieces.
3. Cut the ginger into smaller pieces after peeling it.
4. Squeeze the orange, carrot, and ginger juice through a juicer. If you don't have a juicer, you can still make juice in a blender and then strain it.
5. Give the juice a vigorous stir to blend the flavours after it has been extracted.
6. If preferred, pour the orange carrot ginger juice over ice right away. Before serving, you can also let it cool in the refrigerator.

You are welcome to change the ingredient amounts to fit your own tastes. In addition, you can add some ice cubes or dilute the juice with a little water if you think it's too thick before serving.

Savour the orange carrot ginger juice you made yourself!

VERDANT LEMONADE

How to prepare verdant lemonade.

Component:
-4 peeled kiwi slices and one and a half tablespoons of simple syrup
-half a cup of lime juice
-1/4 cup lime cordial or limeade
-Slices of kiwis or limes as garnish

Direction:
1. Compile the components.
2. In a cocktail shaker, muddle the kiwi and simple syrup.
3. Include the limeade, ice, and lemonade.
Give it a good shake IV. Strain into a highball glass with ice.
4. Add a lime wedge or kiwi slice as a garnish.
5. Present and savour.

Facts about Nutrition (per serving)
341 Calorie, 86g Carbs,
1g Fat, and 3g Protein

Advantages:
1. aid in weight control
2. aid in lowering the risk of cancer
    perhaps beneficial for oral diseases
3. Skin-beneficial and capable of controlling hypertension

4. Prevention of Kidney Stones
5. Helpful for Infection of the Throat
6. Beneficial for Hair
7. Enhance digestion
8. Promotes cardiac health.

GINGER JUICE, LEMON, AND CUCUMBER

How to Prepare Ginger-Lemon Cucumber Water.

Step-by-Step Guide:

1. Get the ingredients ready: Under running water, rinse the cucumber, lemons, and ginger. Cut the cucumbers and lemons into slices, and cut and peel the ginger root.

2. Boil the water to infuse the ginger. Pour the boiling water over the prepared ginger in a heat-resistant glass pitcher or other handy container. Steep for thirty to one hour, or until it's quite warm—ideally chilly. To extract the beneficial components from ginger, heat is required. Cold water doesn't work that well.

3. Mix everything together: Add the cucumber and lemon slices to the cooled water. Fill the pitcher to the brim with cold water, making sure all of the ingredients are submerged.

4. Rest: Allow the flavours and nutrients to seep into the water by letting the combination infuse for at least two hours in the refrigerator.

5. Serve: Transfer the infusion of water into a glass via a strainer or pour, savouring its crisp flavour and health advantages.

When To Sip

When you wake up, right before a meal, right before bed, and right before exercise are the greatest times to consume it.

Nutrition:
 1 **cup serving size**; 10.7kcal of **calories**; 0.1g of **protein**; 6.4 mg of **sodium**; 81.9 mg of **potassium**; 0.2g of **sugar**; 1.2 **IU of vitamin** A; 25.7 mg of **vitamin C;** 2 mg of **calcium**; and 1.2 mg of **iron**.

Advantages
1.Encourages Drinking Water
3.Enhances Gastrointestinal Protection and Function 2. Promotes Weight Loss
4.Aids in the body's waste removal 5. Has anti-inflammatory and antioxidant qualities
6. Strengthens Immunity
7. Encourages Skin Health.

APPLE JUICE AND BEETROOT

This smoothie with apples and beets can be made as follows:

Components:
-One bunch of spinach
-removed two apples' seeds and stalks
-half a lemon, peeled and seeded.

Direction:

1.Rinse all ingredients thoroughly and, if needed, cut them to suit your juicer's feed chute.

2.After adding all the ingredients to your juicer, process and swirl to mix.

3.Serve immediately, either with or without ice.

Juice made from beetroot and apples provides a number of health and weight loss advantages. First off, both ingredients are high in fibre and low in calories, which helps with weight management by encouraging feelings of fullness and consuming fewer calories overall.

This juice's high fibre content promotes gut health and facilitates digestion, which improves nutritional absorption. In addition, the natural sugars in apples offer a consistent supply of energy, which lowers cravings for harmful snacks and helps to keep blood sugar levels stable.

Antioxidants abound in beetroot, especially betalains, which have anti-inflammatory qualities and may aid in the fight against oxidative stress. This may lower the chance of developing chronic illnesses and improve general well-being.

Vitamin C, potassium, folate, and other vital vitamins and minerals are provided by the combination of beetroot and apple, supporting a range of body functions. These nutrients are essential for sustaining good skin, a robust immune system, and cardiovascular health.

Moreover, beetroot has nitrates, which have been connected to better exercise tolerance and endurance. Drinking this drink on a regular basis may increase physical activity and support weight loss attempts.

It's crucial to remember that, even though apple juice and beetroot can be beneficial additions to a healthy lifestyle, for best effects, a balanced diet and frequent exercise are always recommended. Before making any big dietary changes, always get medical advice, especially if you have any underlying medical concerns.

COCONUT JUICE WITH CABANA

Coconut Cabana Juice is a tropical drink that usually blends several fruits with the refreshing taste of coconut.

Ingredients: -
- Coconut milk or water
- Pineapple juice
- Pureed or juiced mangos
- Lime juice
-Cubes of ice

Direction:

1. Put the mango juice (or puree), pineapple juice, and coconut water (or coconut milk) in a blender in equal portions. You can change the precise amounts to fit your taste preferences.
2. Add a squeeze of lime juice for a tart taste.
3. Place several ice cubes in the blender and process until thoroughly mixed and foamy.
4. Taste the mixture and, if necessary, adjust the flavours. To make it taste lighter, use more coconut water; to make it taste sweeter, add more mango juice.
5. Fill glasses with the Coconut Cabana Juice after you're happy with the flavour.
6. If desired, garnish with a wedge of pineapple or a slice of lime.
7. Pour chilled and savour your delightful, tropical Coconut Cabana Juice.

EASY CITRUS MIX

A tasty and refreshing supplement to your weight loss journey can be a breezy citrus combination. Because citrus fruits are high in fibre and low in calories, you can feel content and full after eating less calories. They also contain a lot of vitamins and minerals that are good for general health.

This is a straightforward recipe for a light citrus blend:

Ingredients:
 - One orange - One grapefruit
- One lemon
- One lime
- Mint leaves, fresh (optional)
- Ice cubes, if desired

Guidelines:
1. Wash each and every fruit to get rid of any residue or debris.
2. Cut the orange, lime, grapefruit, and lemon into thin wedges or rounds.
3. To release the flavour of a few fresh mint leaves, if desired, crush them lightly.
4. Place the mint leaves and the sliced citrus fruits in a big pitcher.
5. Pour water into the pitcher, making sure all the fruits are completely soaked.
6. You can add ice cubes to make it more refreshing if you'd like.
7. Gently stir to mix in the flavours.
8. Before serving, let the mixture soak in the fridge for at least one or two hours. You can let it sit overnight for a more intense flavour.
9. Present the light citrus mixture cold and savour!

You can use this citrus combination to replace sugar-filled or high-calorie drinks with something refreshing when it comes to your weight loss regimen. It's crucial to understand that although this combination can be a helpful supplement to an active lifestyle and a balanced diet, it is not a miracle weight-loss cure. A well-rounded approach to exercise and nutrition, along with consistency, are essential for reaching and keeping a healthy weight.

JICAMA PEAR LIQUID

Jicama and pears are combined to create the delightful and healthful beverage known as jicama pear juice. Jicama is a root vegetable native to Central and South America, commonly referred to as Mexican turnip or yam bean. Its flavour is nutty and slightly sweet, and its texture is crisp. Conversely, pears are juicy and taste slightly sweet.

In order to prepare jicama pear juice, the following ingredients are required:

- One medium jicama
- A pair of mature pears
- Water (as required)
- Ice cubes, if desired
This is a basic recipe for making juice from jicama and pear

Direction:
1. Cut the jicama into small pieces after peeling it.
2. Cut the pears into bits after coreing them.
3. Fill a blender with the jicama and pear pieces.
4. To make blending easier, add a tiny bit of water—roughly 1/4 to 1/2 cup.

5. Blend the mixture until it's fully incorporated and smooth. To change the consistency, you can add extra water if preferred.

6. You can add some ice cubes to the blender and process them until they are smashed and mixed into the juice if you would rather have it cold.

7. After the juice has been mixed, taste it and, if needed, add more pears or water to modify the sweetness or thickness.

8. To get rid of any pulp or fibres, if preferred, strain the juice through a fine-mesh screen.

9. Immediately serve the jicama pear juice by pouring it into glasses.

Benefits:

The nutritional qualities of jicama pear juice's primary constituents make it potentially beneficial in a number of ways. The following are some possible advantages of jicama pear juice:

1. *Hydration*: The high water content of jicama pear juice makes it a hydrating beverage. Drinking enough water is crucial for supporting several body processes and preserving general health.

2. *Rich in Fibre:* Pears and jicama provide great dietary fibre sources. Fibre helps facilitate regular bowel movements, supports a healthy digestive system, and may help avoid constipation. Additionally, it enhances the sensation of fullness, which may help with weight management.

3. *Antioxidant Content:* Rich in antioxidants, pears and jicama help shield the body from

damage caused by dangerous free radicals. Chronic diseases including heart disease and some forms of cancer are linked to a lower risk of chronic illnesses when antioxidants are present.

4. *Vitamin C:* Vitamin C is necessary for collagen synthesis, tissue healing, and a robust immune system. Jicama and pears are good providers of this vitamin. Another antioxidant that promotes general health and shields cells from harm is vitamin C.

5. *Packed with Nutrients*: Jicama pear juice has a high content of potassium, magnesium, folate, and vitamin K, among other vitamins and minerals. These nutrients are necessary for a number of body processes, including supporting heart health, fostering bone health, and preserving a healthy blood pressure.

6. *Weight Management*: The juice of jicama pears is low in fat and calories. For anyone trying to control their weight or add healthier options to their diet, it can be a filling and healthy alternative.

7. *Digestive Health*: By encouraging regular bowel movements and offering prebiotic qualities that support good gut bacteria, the dietary fibre in jicama pear juice can support a healthy digestive tract.

It's crucial to remember that each person's unique diet and lifestyle may have an impact on the particular advantages of jicama pear juice. Before making big dietary changes, it's always a good idea to speak with a medical expert or certified dietitian if you have any specific health issues.

PURPLE FRUITS PEACHES AND PARSLEY

Purple fruits, peaches, and parsley are combined to create purple peach parsley juice, a cool and wholesome drink. This bright juice is made with ease using this recipe:

Ingredients include:
 - Two juicy peaches -
-Two purple plums -
-A handful of fresh parsley leaves
- Water (extra, for uniformity)

Directions:
1. Give the parsley, peaches, and plums a good wash.
2. Remove the pits from the plums and peaches and chop them into smaller pieces.
3. Fill a blender with the plums, peaches, and parsley leaves.
4. Process the mixture at a high speed until it's smooth and thoroughly mixed. You can adjust the consistency by adding a small amount of water if the mixture is too thick.
5. After blending, strain the juice through cheesecloth or a fine-mesh strainer to get rid of any pulp or particles.
6. Fill glasses with the juice, then serve right away.

JUICE OF HONEYDEW APPLE

A delicious drink called honeydew apple juice is created by mixing apple juice with honeydew melon. It's a well-liked option for people who wish to experience a different flavour combination and appreciate fruit drinks.

You'll need fresh honeydew melon and apples to produce honeydew apple juice. To help you get started, consider this easy recipe:

Ingredients:
-1 melon with honeydew.
- Four apples

Instructions:
1. Thoroughly wash the apples and honeydew melon to get rid of any dirt or debris.
2. Scoop out the seeds by cutting the honeydew melon in half. After that, chop the melon into bits and remove the rind.
3. Slice the apples after removing the cores.
4. Put the apple slices and honeydew melon chunks into a juicer.
5. Start the juicer and run it through the fruits until all of the juice is extracted.
6. You can strain the juice to get rid of any pulp or solids if you'd like.

7. Immediately serve the honeydew apple juice over ice, or store it in the refrigerator for later use.

Advantages:
A combination of apple juice and honeydew melon, honeydew apple juice has a number of advantages. The following are a few possible benefits of drinking honeydew apple juice:

1. *Packed with nutrients:* Apples and honeydew melon are both excellent sources of important vitamins, minerals, and antioxidants. Whereas apples offer vitamin C, dietary fibre, and different antioxidants like flavonoids, honeydew melon is a wonderful source of vitamin C, potassium, and dietary fibre.

2. *Hydration*: Because honeydew apple juice has a high water content, it can aid in body hydration. Drinking enough water is essential for supporting several body processes and preserving general health.

3. *Digestive health:* The dietary fibre in apples and honeydew melon can facilitate regular bowel motions and help with digestion. Consuming enough fibre is essential for keeping the digestive tract in good working order.

4. *Antioxidant qualities*: Antioxidants, which shield your cells from damage by dangerous substances known as free radicals, are present in both honeydew melon and apples. Antioxidants contribute to general well-being by lowering the risk of chronic illnesses.

5. *Immune support*: The vitamin C concentration of honeydew apple juice helps to support the immune system. It is well known that vitamin C supports immune function and aids in the body's ability to fight off infections.

6. *Refreshing flavour*: Honeydew apple juice is naturally sweet and refreshing, making it a fun and healthful substitute for sugar-filled drinks. It might be a fantastic choice for people seeking a tasty non-alcoholic beverage.

Keep in mind that honeydew apple juice still contains natural sugars and calories, so drink it in moderation.

LEMON JUICE WITH MANGO WATER

Juicy watermelons and ripe mangoes are blended to create the delightful and refreshing beverage known as mango watermelon juice. The ideal balance of sweetness and tropical tastes is achieved.

Here's a basic recipe you may use to make mango watermelon juice:

***Ingredients*:**

- 4 cups chopped watermelon
 - 2 ripe mangoes - Ice cubes (optional)
- Garnish with fresh mint leaves (optional)

Guidelines:
1. Remove the flesh from the pit of the mangoes by peeling them. Dice the flesh of the mango.
2. Trim the watermelon of any seeds, if needed, and cut into tiny, manageable pieces.
3. Fill a blender with the watermelon and mango chunks.
4. Process the fruits at a high speed in a blender until the mixture is smooth and uniform.
5. To make the juice colder and more refreshing, feel free to add some ice cubes to the blender. Process once more to crush and integrate the ice cubes.
6. Fill glasses with the mango watermelon juice.
7. For an extra touch of freshness and aesthetic appeal, consider adding a sprig of fresh mint leaves to the rim of each glass.
8. Pour the juice right away and savor!

You can modify this recipe to suit your personal preferences. If you would like more sweetness, you can add a teaspoon of honey or a squeeze of lime juice for a tangy touch.

PINK GRAPE FRUIT DELIGHT

The vivid and tangy flavours of pink grapefruit are highlighted in Pink Grapefruit Delight, a wonderful and refreshing dessert or snack. The following is a basic recipe for Pink Grapefruit Delight

Ingredients:
 - One cup of whipped cream or whipped topping
- Two large pink grapefruits
- Two teaspoons (optional) of honey or maple syrup
- Optional garnish of fresh mint leaves

Direction:
1. The first step is to cut the pink grapefruits in half lengthwise. With a sharp knife, carefully cut off the fruit's outer peel and the membrane that divides its segments. Eliminate any seeds as well.
2. After placing the grapefruit segments in a basin, squeeze any residual membrane juice into the bowl. Keep the juice for later.
3. Use whipped topping or cream that has been beaten until soft peaks form in a another bowl. You can fold in some honey or maple syrup to sweeten the whipped cream if you'd like.
4. Place a layer of grapefruit segments at the bottom of serving cups or bowls. To enhance the flavour of the segments, drizzle a small amount of the conserved grapefruit juice over them.
5. Next, cover the grapefruit segments entirely with a layer of whipped cream or whipped topping.
6. Continue layering, adding additional grapefruit segments, dripping juice, and finishing with whipped cream until the glasses or bowels are full.
7. To finish, place a dollop of whipped cream on top and, if preferred, garnish with fresh mint leaves.

8. Place the Pink Grapefruit Delight in the refrigerator for a minimum of one hour to allow the flavours to combine and the dessert to cool.
9. Present cold and savour!

Citrus enthusiasts will appreciate Pink Grapefruit Delight, a light and delightful dessert. The pleasant contrast of flavours is created when the creamy whipped cream and the acidic grapefruit combine.

FRESCA MELON AQUA

Because of its moisturising qualities and low calorie content, melon agua fresca might be a beneficial supplement to a diet plan for weight loss. Melons naturally contain a lot of water and little calories, so eating them can help you feel satiated and full without consuming too many calories. A weight-loss-focused variation of the recipe is provided here:

Ingredients:
– 1 ripe melon (honeydew or cantaloupe)
– 4 cups water
- Stevia, or similar sugar substitute without calories, according to taste (optional)
• Ice cubes
- Fresh mint leaves (garnish if desired)

Direction:
1. Slice the melon in half, then take out the seeds. Remove the meat and chop it into pieces.

2. Fill a blender with the chopped melon.

3. Fill the blender with water and process Up Until the mixture is the consistency of a smooth liquid.

4. Optional: Strain the mixture through a fine-mesh strainer to get rid of any pulp or seeds if you'd like it smoother.

5. Give the mixture a taste. If you think it needs more sweetness, you can use a tiny bit of stevia or another natural zero-calorie sweetener. Remember that melons are naturally sweet, so you might get away with using less sweetener.

6. Place the melon Fresca in the fridge to chill for at least half an hour.

7. When serving time comes, put ice cubes in glasses.

Pour the Melon Agua Fresca over the ice cubes once it has cooled down.

9. You can optionally garnish with fresh mint leaves. Mix thoroughly and savour your calorie-free and revitalising Melon Agua Fresca!

Remember that for effective and long-lasting weight loss, it's crucial to concentrate on general good eating habits and frequent physical activity. Melon Agua Fresca can be a healthy complement to a weight loss plan.

DRINKABLE PINEAPPLE LAVENDER

Pineapple lavender juice combines the fragrant, floral notes of lavender with the tropical sweetness of pineapple to create a delightful and unique beverage.

For your reference, here is a basic recipe:

-Four glasses of water
-one ripe pineapple
-one dried lavender bud
-and your favourite sweetener (optional)

Direction:
1. After peeling and cored the pineapple, cut it into thin slices.
2. In a blender or juicer, combine the pineapple chunks with water. Mix until smooth, blending the ingredients.
3. Empty the pineapple mixture into a pitcher or container.
4. Add the dried lavender buds to the pitcher, stirring well.
5. Put the mixture in the refrigerator for at least an hour to allow the flavours to mingle.
6. Following the predetermined infusion time, strain the liquid to extract the lavender buds.
7. You can optionally add sugar after tasting the juice. The honey or agave syrup can be replaced with any other sweetener of your choosing.
8. Toss in the sweetener and stir thoroughly.
Take pleasure in the ice-cold pineapple-lavender juice!

Naturally! Pineapple Lavender Juice is a delightful concoction of tastes that offers a unique twist on traditional fruit drinks.

Some further details and benefits for each element are as follows:

1.Pineapple: Pineapples are tropical fruits that are prized for their sweet and acidic taste. Bromelain, an enzyme that breaks down food, and a lot of vitamin C are all found in it. By contributing a cold, tropical flavour, pineapple balances the lavender's floral notes in the juice.

2. *Lavender*: This herb has a slightly sweet, flowery flavour and is very fragrant. It is often used in confections, teas, and other culinary uses. Lavender is commonly used to promote rest and reduce tension because to its calming properties. To offset the richness of the fruit, lavender adds a subtle floral flavour and scent to pineapple lavender juice.

3. *Health Benefits*: - Antioxidant strength and collagen production depend on vitamin C, which is found in large quantities in pineapples.

An anti-inflammatory and perhaps digestive chemical found in pineapples is called bromelain.
Because lavender may help promote relaxation and reduce anxiety, it is commonly used for these purposes.
The antibacterial and antioxidant properties of lavender are believed to exist.

A spicy, energising juice made with pineapple and lavender is excellent served straight up or as a base for other beverages. Test varying additions like as ginger, lemon juice, or mint leaves to further enhance the flavour profile.

It tastes best when consumed fresh, just like any other homemade juice, and has the most nutritious benefit.

<u>CONCLUSION</u>

Juicing can be a useful strategy for novices looking to lose weight. It provides a practical means of consuming an assortment of fruits and vegetables in liquid form, offering necessary nutrients and lowering caloric intake. Juicing should, therefore, be used into a well-rounded and long-term weight loss strategy.

For newbies wishing to include weight loss juicing recipes in their practice, keep in mind these important takeaways:

1. *Ingredients high in nutrients*: The main goal of weight loss juicing recipes should be to use a range of fruits and vegetables that are high in antioxidants, vitamins, and minerals. Leafy greens like kale and spinach as well as fruits like oranges, berries, and apples are examples.

2. *Calorie control:* Juicing can aid with calorie restriction, but it's important to be aware of the juices' total calorie count. Certain fruits, like mangos and bananas, have a lot of natural sugars and can add a lot of calories. Finding the right balance between taste and calorie restriction is crucial.

3. *Portion control:* When using juices for weight loss, be mindful of portion amounts. Even though they might not contain many calories, eating too much of them can nonetheless cause weight gain. The key is moderation.

4. *Balanced diet:* Whole foods shouldn't be completely replaced by juice. It's critical to include a range of other nutrient-dense foods in your diet, including whole grains, lean proteins, and healthy

fats. Although it can boost your overall vitamin intake, juicing shouldn't be your only source of nutrition.

5. *Exercise*: Juicing by itself might not be a long-term solution for weight loss. It is crucial to incorporate it with consistent exercise to increase metabolism, burn fat, and gain muscle. To achieve the best weight loss outcomes, try walking, running, swimming, or strength training.

6. *Long-term sustainability*: Although juicing is a helpful weight-loss strategy, not everyone will find it to be practical or sustainable over the long term. Long-term solid food restriction can have detrimental effects on general health and result in dietary shortages. It's crucial to speak with a qualified nutritionist or healthcare provider to make sure you're getting the nutrition you need.

Never forget that there is no one-size-fits-all method for losing weight; it is a progressive process. A healthy lifestyle that incorporates a balanced diet, consistent exercise, and long-lasting habits might benefit greatly from the inclusion of juicing.

Daily Juicing Remark

Day	Recipe	Remark